Yoga,
My Bed & M.E.

Donna Owens

ॐ Contents ॐ

My purpose is to support and help people
feel brighter, happier and healthier through yoga.

ॐ About This Book ॐ

I know how difficult it is to feel human, calm and content all at once with M.E. struggling everyday with simple tasks, juggling family, work and play. I also know how exercise can be a big "no no" to a lot of people (depending on limits, symptoms and severity). Sometimes you can't get out of bed. Your body is heavy, sore and tight, yet your mind is fine and wants to do something. It's like a puppy wanting to play while your body wants a nap or the other way around or where your brain feels like it's been removed, but your body is twitchy and restless.

It can be frustrating and depressing. People without the condition, don't "get" it because they can't see our "wounds". It's hard (and energy draining) to constantly try to explain to people about the condition. It can be heart-breaking trying to keep "up" with family and friends. Even worse is if the people closest to you don't show and give you the support that you need, because "you look ok!"

If you're a chronic fatigue warrior, who is looking for gentle and calming exercise, then this book is your guide. A guide to give your body and mind some love. This is where yoga comes in. This is a yoga "workout" that you don't have to get out of bed for, no yoga pants needed, just your favourite pjs.

Although this book is related to M.E. the illness close to my heart, it's designed to help anyone who suffers from fatigue, muscle aches and pains. People who are bed or housebound. People who want to relax, stretch out aches, to gain some energy and blood flow to the body during the day, but who also want help to relax the body for a healthy sleep. This book can also help people with mild depression or anxiety issues, as it helps to calm the mind. You see, yoga is for anyone who is willing to try a new approach.

This book is split into sections: Yoga Poses: A breakdown of poses which you can pick, practise and hold to suit you when and where you need it. Yoga Sequences: Simple and recommended routines - one for muscle awakening to do in the mornings - one for muscle relaxation to do before bed or meditation - a quick pick me up routine and one for bad M.E. days. Lastly, there is a breathing and meditation chapter to help you in times of stress and to help your mental clarity. Do the routines to suit your condition, your limits and preferences. Pick and choose poses that you feel help you more and just relax into them for as long as is comfortable for you. Do the whole "workout", make it longer or shorter depending on how you feel, and we all feel different each day so don't force your body (or mind) if it doesn't want to do yoga or get in a certain pose any day. Your body will guide you where it wants to go, respect it. As with any workout programme please get medical advice before starting and embarking on any physical activity, especially if you suffer from heart trouble, eye problems, chronic back issues, high blood pressure or are / think you are pregnant.

Above all, listen to your body. I am just a guide. Your body is your teacher. I wrote this book through experience and with love. I'm not a medical expert and far from a pretzel yogi master. I wanted to help, and to share first-hand what worked for me during my M.E. battle. To share what helped me cope through hours of endless muscle pains, sleepless nights and panic attacks. I wanted to support others who are battling as I was. My advice to you: believe in yourself.

I hope this book is helpful to you, your body and mind. That it enables you to gain an insight into yoga and how it can be adapted to help many conditions physically, emotionally and mentally.

Namaste

Donna

www.donnayogagirl.com

ॐ About Me ॐ

As a yoga teacher and a M.E. warrior, I know all about the pros of yoga and the cons of M.E. (I don't like the word sufferer. We are all in fact warriors who are doing a remarkable job with the difficulties we face).

M.E. was not something I openly talked about for many years, mainly due to the lack of understanding M.E. had when I was first ill. I went through the nightmare as a teenager and didn't want to waste my precious energy on repeatedly explaining something over and over to people who didn't want to believe it was a real illness.

I became ill at 12, following a winter virus, which never left. At my worst, I could barely walk, shuffling was about it (Hey! There's a song about that now!). I found it hard to talk, eat, write or to keep my eyes open. I felt like a stone Zombie, suffering with severe muscle pain, sickness, tiredness, restlessness and mental issues amongst other symptoms. I was in tears during most of my teenage years. I couldn't deal with noise and crowds very well. When I did manage to go out, I felt as though I was a power source for everyone's "hyper" energy. Everyone seemed to be on fast forward and loud mode while I was on mute and slow motion. When I managed to get to school (which got less and less as time went on) I couldn't understand why all my classmates were so hyper and talking so loud. It hurt my head and ears and made me feel spaced out.

I was envious that they seemed to do everything with a spring in their step and I didn't even have energy to move a finger. I wanted to fit in, have energy and be like them. I over pushed my energy levels numerous times trying to be "normal" and liked. I wasn't very popular and regularly got some stick for always "pretending to be ill" and "always being off school". That resulted in mild depression. I remember in the 90`s being told "you`re just 13! What have YOU got to be depressed about!?" or it was brushed off as a "moody teen" phase.

I felt scared, isolated, in pain, depressed and worse of all I didn't know why this was happening to me and didn't know what it was.

When I had a "good day" I pushed myself doing too much as I felt I had to prove to people I was normal. I wanted to be normal! I would walk to school, I would laugh and run around at break time, but soon after I was back in bed and stuck there for days or weeks on end. It was a constant exhausting cycle.

It`s hard enough to be a young teenager, with all the physical and emotional changes that the body goes through without the bad symptoms of M.E. on top. Teen years are the hardest, biggest, supposedly the most exciting part of growing up. So much happens, so much is learnt and experienced, making friends, bonding, good times and lessons, and I missed it all from being asleep, in pain, in bed or house bound for months on end.

M.E. suffered from a major lack of understanding back in the early 90`s. My doctor at the time (after my illness was dragging on) didn't believe in M.E. She stopped giving out sick notes and made it out as though I was the "naughty kid" who didn't want to go school. School and social welfare involvement didn't help my illness with their stern talks. Forcing me out of bed, making me go to school. I would walk to school as we didn't have a car. It was about a 40-minute walk from home to school. I would get to school, only for the teachers to send me home at lunchtime, because I was ill, white as a sheet, not focusing, and feeling dizzy. This then got the welfare officer banging at my door the next day asking why I wasn't in school again.

I got so scared that I would hide under my bed every time the doorbell went or a car pulled up in the street, in case it was someone coming around to shout at me. I was missing more and more of school, which made it harder to go back. School never sent any homework for me, or tried to help with my studying. I missed so much that the days I did go in I was lost and way behind and couldn't take part in most of the lessons. Anxiety mixed with depression kicked in along with everything else. I didn't realize I was suffering from anxiety and panic attacks until many years later. I actually thought it was me being silly over small things and I didn't link the two together. (I still suffer badly with anxiety which is a challenge in itself).

I cried A LOT! But that made me even more tired than I was already. Some nights no matter how much I wanted to cry, I was just too exhausted to sob my heart out. Everyone said I was fine, being lazy or a sulking teen. I saw lots of different doctors, went to many appointments, and received mixed advice and diagnoses of what was wrong. They finally sent me to a local hospital to see a specialist. Yet more hospital appointments followed to be still told they couldn't find anything wrong over and over again. I had sooo many blood tests, that I could have stocked Dracula up nicely for a month. It was like a broken record for over two years. It's not a surprise that people see many different medical experts before they get a diagnosis. While I understand that diagnosis of the illness is complicated, fatigue being the most common symptom in M.E. and a million other illnesses which need to be ruled out along the way, it's still a long and exhausting road for someone who is constantly exhausted. I was finally diagnosed when I was 14, following a long two-year battle with doctors, hospitals and my school. It took many appointments before one doctor at the hospital actually agreed and said the words "IT'S M.E.", after we had questioned him to actually get him to say it. It was a relief. If I am honest I can't remember much of the talking at any of the appointments. Everything was and still is a blur. Once diagnosed, I can't remember getting any aftercare, no "what's next", no "let us help you", no pills they just seemed to have sent me away to get on with it.

After my M.E. was confirmed school was still rather horrid, I suffered panic attacks regularly and missed much time and work, let alone being able to write, stay awake or concentrate on anything. I have no idea how it came about, but my family with help from the hospital managed to get me a private home tutor a couple of mornings a week and I left school permanently. This was more of a relief to me than the hospital diagnosis. The pure stress of school and panic over the 2 years was a major factor in making my symptoms a 100 times worse and any recovery impossible.

The home tutoring meant I could fit "lessons" in around the times and days when I was "brighter". My memory was so bad; I couldn't retain information. I struggled with putting a sentence together. Concentration was nowhere to be seen. I couldn't write very well; my hand would feel like it was turning to stone as I tried to write. We only did (more like tried to do) basic maths, English, life skills and art as I enjoyed that. I still struggle with brain fog and feel brain dead if I'm overtired. My facial muscles drop and I start slurring words (without touching a drop) and don't even ask me to do maths in my head!

It was a long slow road, but I was learning slowly to relax now I knew what it was (kind of) and was no longer in a constant scared state over school, doctors and thinking it was all in my head. I could learn to deal with the illness myself and find out what I could and couldn't do. It was a lot of trial and error most of the time. A lot of fall-backs and frustration, but by being gentle with myself and body, in time I worked it out.

M.E. is a life- changing illness, even when recovery has improved. The internet wasn't available when I was a teenager, so there was no online social media to stay in contact with people, to meet people with similar stories or Google for help when you wanted information or to research symptoms (always the wrong idea to do!). Support groups were few and far. You had to get out to a meeting environment, a tad difficult when bed bound! Books or easy access to knowledge about the condition were few and far between also. I found one book in a local bookshop many moons ago and at 14 with my part time brain, I didn't understand it or read it all until a few years ago. At that time, mobile phones were bricks and I obviously didn't have one, let alone a smartphone with everything at the touch of a button keeping me socially active and able to access support.

All the time, being ill made me feel alone, I hardly had or saw any friends. I felt depressed and lost a lot of the time. But, the one thing I did find was myself. I still prefer being alone than in a houseful of people. I'm still sensitive to noise, especially lots of different chattering around me. I love peace and quiet. I can tune into myself, my needs and wants better. It took years of self-learning about myself, my body and its limits to slowly control the illness and work around it, so I could have a life.

I got into fashion magazines and makeup at 13. It took my mind off the illness and into hobbies. Collecting makeup, copying the "in" looks and designing styles, I was always arty and wanted a career in something creative, and I found it in makeup. I put my heart and soul into practicing, reading and getting great at it. My tutor worked makeup / hair projects into our English, maths and life skills lessons, teaching me what would help me achieve being a makeup artist. At 16, I enrolled in a hairdressing and beauty course at my local college. Scared, as I had no entry GCSEs results and had no idea how my health would behave, I had at least worked hard for 2 years with a portfolio that I made to show my passion and determination for my career choice. With an interview I got a place on the course. My teachers were more supportive of me and my illness during the 3 years I was there than any doctor had been in the past. I had a social life. I had purpose and I was learning all of which made me feel accomplished. I still had flare ups but they were controllable and college let me have the time I needed to recover when I needed it.

I worked for myself once qualified. I did try a couple of jobs in salons, but it was all too much after just a few weeks. The long hours and M.E. didn't mix. I did mobile hairdressing and worked the days and hours to fit in with M.E. up until 2002 when I became pregnant with my daughter. Pregnancy was a challenge. For the first 4 months I was bed ridden with M.E. and feeling sick. From 5 months plus, I was sick, couldn't eat and felt horrid. No blooming pregnancy for this mamma! I hired a yoga teacher to help me while pregnant, mainly just to make sure I was doing yoga correctly while carrying the baby and to help with labour. It must have worked, because to me, the labour was the easiest and quickest part of the whole 9 months. Although the months of being sick caught up with me and I was underweight at just 7 stone after giving birth.

After my daughter was born, it was a whirlwind of change. We moved from Devon to Lancashire when she was just 4 months old. M.E. didn't have time for a look in, although I was very lucky with a quiet, happy baby. I spent my days resting, yoga breathing and cuddling. I put my daughter and my health first so I could be the best mum I could and I wasn't going let M.E. take over.

As time went on, I trained as a fashion makeup artist and worked successfully for over 10 years in Lancashire doing bridal, photo shoots and magazine work. Still working for myself so I could balance work, motherhood and illness, I had a few bad spells through the years. Relationships broke down and I felt lonely again. My illness was being mis-understood by people who were meant to be close. I felt people didn't register that I needed space, lie-ins, rest days and help. I was looked upon as lazy and moody. I was unhappy, ill health came back leading to more hospital appointments where nothing was found. I was homesick, depressed and wanted more from life so that my daughter would grow up happy. So I made the biggest decision I ever made in 2007 and moved back down to Devon to be nearer help, family and the quiet countryside. I knew my M.E. would hit with a break-up and stress and my work would suffer as there's no call for makeup in Devon, but I had to do what was right in my heart. I had a new lease of life, after a few months of M.E. relapse, depression and anxiety. I learnt to drive. My daughter was a constant smiling ray of sunshine at school. I got my friends back and lived for a while, something I never did as a young lady because of M.E. I carried on with makeup for a few years travelling for the work around the country. Over time my passion died and the travelling tired me. I didn't like being so far away from my daughter. What if anything happened to her at school? Anxiety was bubbling away under the surface, but this was my job. What would I do if I didn't do makeup? I had worked so hard battling M.E. and fighting to make it a success for years, it seemed wrong to just throw my progress down the drain.

My ultimate dream was to teach and open a makeup school. The opportunity to teach fell into my lap in 2012. I hadn't had a bad M.E. relapse for years and it was one day a week so I went for it. 9 weeks in and bang! I ran straight into the M.E. brick wall. With my anxiety levels at an all-new high. I couldn't leave the house, or leave my bed and I felt like that 14-year-old girl all over again, wanting to hide under the bed. This time I had a daughter to stay strong for. I didn't want her to worry or be scared and suffer. Not to mention having to provide for her. I felt stupid. I was a grown woman! So why was I feeling like a helpless child? I ended up on anti-depressants a few times. Some made me feel worse, sick or emotionless. I wasn't sleeping. I didn't know what to do. I felt I was letting people down, useless and alone again. It was dragging on. I prayed for something to happen or for something to help me from this dark hole. I remember at 6am on a Monday morning I jumped awake. I had a lightbulb moment! I called mum instantly and said, "Yoga! I'm going to do yoga for a living!" Why didn't I think of this before?! I didn't know what yoga path I was meant to be on back then, but it felt like home.

I had been doing "yoga" throughout the illness in my teens. I didn't know I was doing yoga. I was just stretching and trying to ease the pain. I discovered what yoga really was when I was 18, while trying to find something to help me with the chronic muscle aches in my legs. I needed something to help make my body feel alive instead of like a pile of heavy bones making a permanent nest in my bed.

When you're crying in pain most nights you'll try anything once, right? Of course, I was still very weak, most of the yoga books I found weren't clear, were too much for my body or were too hard to understand with concentration issues. Videos (Yes!! Good old videos, before YouTube, DVDs and Blu-rays) were all too much for my condition and were aimed at fitness more than health or were too old-fashioned and rather off-putting.

I overdid doing yoga many times, pushing myself through videos and workouts which I thought would do me good, but which left me bed ridden afterwards. I learnt I had to go slowly and build my own yoga up.

I picked certain yoga poses from a book. Something I could keep close to hand that I could flick through and which I felt would help when and where I was aching the most that day or night (legs, calves and hamstrings every time). I just held the poses for as long as possible, (I did the Seated Forward Bend a lot) covered up in duvet, cuddling a pillow and often dozed off in the posture waiting until I felt the pain and tension wash away from my legs.

Even if it was 1 pose for 2 minutes or for up to an hour it helped, not for long, but it gave me enough time to let my mind and muscles relax. I constantly found myself doing two yoga poses over and over again. The Seated Wide Angle Forward Bend, and as mentioned the Seated Forward Bend (both found in this book with details of their benefits). I did yoga when and as I needed. I didn't have a mat. I didn't have yoga time. I didn't even do a 20 minute "workout". I wasn't a yogi nor did I do it every day. I just knew that stretching helped.

I have always come back to yoga throughout the years, through M.E. relapses, broken hearts, dislocated knee, pregnancy, operations and single motherhood as I know it works for me. Though I wouldn't call it real yoga in the beginning, more like musical statues, without the music.... or dancing. Just lying there in a pose while reading, watching television, colouring or mainly snoozing.

Now, fast forward about 15 years, and I'm suddenly in my 30's (boo) and a yoga teacher (yay!) I still suffer from M.E. (more boos) and I still use yoga to help with muscle pains in the body. I still lie on my bed holding poses. This time, holding them as I nose through my smartphone, messages or type this book. This is how *Yoga, My Bed & M.E.* started. I always had half a book written about my story. As I became a yoga teacher, I tried different types of yoga. I knew I didn't want to hold classes, so I did healing yoga with clients. Power yoga became popular with women wanting to lose weight and tone up. I had to space the clients and had to avoid M.E. days. It brought in money for summer, but went quiet in the winter. I still felt something was missing from my business and I started to get a bit down again, why wasn't this working? Yoga is my path, I knew it! I took myself away from people and technology and I wrote notes, putting my fears, limits and dreams down. It soon became clear my path was to help other M.E. warriors through yoga.

That's when I decided to set up *Yoga, My Bed & M.E.* guides, online yoga and M.E. support. I made a promise to myself to finish this book and reach out to the many people who need a caring hand throughout their battle with the illness.

To this day, I'm still learning and facing new challenges. M.E. is now my business partner, it is also my guide to health and happiness, despite its horrid ways. It tells me when enough is enough. It stops me and brings me back to myself and my roots. It gives me the head space and time I need to see and feel where my life is going, decide what to do and to notice the beauty and what's going on around me.

ॐ About M.E. Illness ॐ

It`s a shame with so many warriors and families caring for people, that still a lot of people aren't aware of the illness, have limited knowledge about it or still don't believe in it. On the plus side, there are also so many more that do, and now, thanks to social media and the internet there is alot of online information and also groups, associations, books and help. Support is available to everyone with a touch of a button.

So here's a breakdown of some M.E. facts and symptoms. I`m keeping it light and breezy as I`m not a medical expert on the illness and this is just from my own personal illness, knowledge and experience. There is no medical jargon so it`s easily understood and simple. It also means I don't have to try to spell long fancy words.

M.E. stands for Myalgic Encephalomyelitis (Damn there`s the first long word).

Over 250,000 people are estimated to suffer from that long fancy word in the UK alone. Everyone suffers differently and the symptoms vary a lot, which makes it harder for doctors to diagnose. They have to go through an elimination process of other illnesses before a diagnosis can be confirmed.

Very few people make a full recovery from the illness. Many will suffer from relapses throughout their lives, triggered by illness or physical / mental stress.

The deep cause of M.E. is still unknown. It is linked to adrenal gland fatigue, the glands which are meant to help the body deal with stress. M.E. attacks the immune system, which as we know is the body's defence system against foreign bodies and illnesses. As the immune system is in a constant battle with the problems we face, we constantly feel run down and can suffer with sore throats, sickness, swollen glands and flu-type symptoms.

The illness usually begins from a viral infection (colds, flu). Mine started when I came down with flu, which went onto glandular fever, and never got better. Most people who suffer from the illness were active, busy and happy people before being struck down. For many people this leads to a feeling of helplessness and frustration. M.E. also attacks the central nervous system which in turn leads to abnormal brain functioning and problems such as brain fog, lack of concentration, dizziness and varying extreme body temperatures. It can also be triggered by a stressful event in the person's life, such as an accident, operation or personal grief.

M.E. has a wide range of symptoms. These include chronic fatigue and unexplained tiredness from simple mental and/or physical tasks, which don't go away after rest. There may be sleep disturbances, feeling too hot or extremely cold, painful muscles and joints, headaches, sensitivity to light and sound, dizziness, poor memory, and concentration and panic attacks. These symptoms which can last several months at a time are just a few of those that can occur. It's a life of a constant cycle of relapse and remission for the warrior.

The symptoms' severity varies between warriors greatly. It affects the whole person physically, mentally and emotionally for very long periods of time, and we're talking years sometimes. Some people have been house or bed-bound or having to use wheelchairs during these long periods of time.

It interferes with lives and makes day to day functioning nearly impossible. Relapses can hit sufferers if they push themselves too much, do too much or if they get hit with an illness or stress. Relapses can be brought on even if they have improved in health for a while, for months or years. It has taken me years to learn to cope and pace my body with the illness and life, and even more years to learn to cope with the neurological side of the illness (writing this book and lifestyle changes have brought on the need and want to better my battered brain).

So, the first big main symptom is fatigue. Total mental and physical fatigue from just simple everyday tasks. The type of tiredness that would give Sleeping Beauty a run for her money....and win! And after those 100 plus years of sleep, you're still tired and feel like you haven't slept a wink the whole time. Yes, I know we ALL get tired, I get tired and drained trying to explain to narrow minded people that it's not everyday tiredness. I can't "just get over it", I'm not "lazy". I go to bed at a good time and it's not an excuse to avoid doing something.

This is tiredness like you've gone 100mph straight into a brick wall. Tiredness that takes over your whole body. Tiredness which makes you bed-ridden for days, months or years. Tiredness where you can't walk or hold your toothbrush to clean your teeth. Tiredness where you really are too tired to talk and your words start to slur, you are too tired to eat and it hurts to lift your arm to feed yourself and even to chew food. It can involve feeling so sick, as though you have just run a marathon without training for it. Yet explaining it to some people is just a waste of vital energy when most reply with "that's a bit exaggerated, don't you think?"

At 13 trying to explain this to the medical world obviously put me in the "she's got an over active imagination", "issues", "a cry for attention?" group. It can be a very lonely illness and is often ignored.

I found I couldn't stay awake for long. I could have slept all night and day. My body hated (and still does) alarms, being suddenly woken up and early calls. Forcing myself to be awake and up sent me back to bed by noon or if I couldn't rest / nap and had to push myself, I would be back in bed for days or weeks afterwards. The overpowering wave of tiredness is draining both physically and mentally to the body. It is all too easy to try and push through the tiredness in the hope we'll shake it off as the days go by. It isn't the case with M.E. Chances are as the day goes on, the body gets worse not better. You become clumsy. It starts to feel like you're slowly turning to stone, everything goes into slow motion, walking, talking, tasks. It takes all your energy to keep your eyes open and keep your facial muscles up and not feeling like your face is melting down to the ground, which then results in bad headaches.

With body fatigue, comes body pain. Flu-type body pain that can last and last. Heavy arms and legs that you can't lift or move because they ache so much. Muscle pain brought me to tears numerous times over the years and not knowing how to make it stop. Also restless painful legs and not knowing what to do with them. The feeling like an elephant had sat on my lap waiting for a bedtime story, yet at the same time, my legs felt like they were moving and jumping at record speed and tiring me out and making my legs ache more. I experienced joint pain in knees and shoulders, painful swollen lymph nodes in the neck and stomach, and the constant 24/7 dull ache all over that made it impossible to know what to do with myself.

This is why I started yoga all those years ago and why I still love yoga to this day. It helps to move and stretch out every part of my body. To relax the muscles, release stiffness, ward off headaches and keep my mind focused on what I am doing, how my body is feeling and how I am emotionally. It helps me to feel, if even if it`s for a minute, that I am in a happy smiling place.

With the tiredness in the body, the brain goes on strike too. M.E. is also a neurological condition which affects mental functioning as it affects the central nervous system. You struggle to focus on things, tasks, reading, writing, talking. The word Zombie comes to mind, and I'm sure I have felt and looked like one many times over the years. Trying to concentrate when over-exhausted physically, is well, bloody hard work! The energy you feel you are using up while you try to take something in is overwhelming. You get frustrated with yourself so you try harder. It`s like trying to move a stone with just the power of your mind. All that focus and nothing. Before you know it, you`re out of battery power and upset with yourself which makes you more tired.

Along with concentration and the attention span being affected, my biggest neuro symptom is still mental blockage. A lot of times I can`t find or spell words, I know what I want to say and type but I just freeze, like I actually know absolutely nothing. I can`t think and actually zone (or Zombie) out and the lights go out in my brain for a few minutes. The harder I try to remember how to spell the word, the emptier my brain goes. I still can`t do maths, not to save my life; the above applies, I get frustrated with numbers and go blank. I do get down when I struggle in front of people who do it from the top of their heads. I've struggled and got upset with myself a number of times trying to help my daughter with her primary school maths homework. I've felt useless, thick and a rubbish parent at times. I can carry on struggling, getting tense and wearing my battery down which could lead to a minor relapse or I can laugh it off and move on, after all we have calculators, don't we?

Loss of memory is another issue for M.E. warriors. Personally, it adds to the emotional side of the illness for me. I forget little things regarding my daughter which people normally remember and treasure, time of birth, weight, first word, the where and when things happened. I can't remember much except her weight, randomly, thanks to my brain taking naps.

So, on top of the physical and mental challenges that affect us, we also have to deal with the emotional difficulties it brings, which is probably the most personal and intimate challenge of them all. I am a firm believer that physical and emotional issues are connected. Both show signs when things go wrong. You can't have one without the other.

My emotional health departed at the age of 4 following the death of my dad. I know it affected me, but I can't remember how I was or my emotions. I didn't know what emotions were and growing up it was very much a locked door. For years I avoided the subject and wouldn't talk about it. I didn't grieve, accept and let it go throughout my childhood. I kept everything inside to protect myself, to avoid looking weak, breaking down or dealing with it. I didn't want pity or to have to answer questions. I'm not saying my dad's death was the root cause of M.E. but I'm sure the heavy invisible sack of emotions I was carrying on my back for all those years didn't help me physically. Along with growing up, hormones, puberty and teenage years all adding their own emotional and physical heaviness to the sack, finally, the sack was too heavy and I crashed.

Emotionally, it's hard to come to terms with the illness. The feeling of being useless, in constant pain, being misunderstood and not being yourself after living a good active life before the illness can bring on depression, grief and anger. At the beginning of the illness I was made more confused, lonely and scared by not knowing what was wrong with me. By the age of 14 I was emotionally hurt by what seemed like everyone not believing that I was ill. I felt I was treated like a toddler a lot of the time, adults talking over me about "my issues" and not listening to (or believing) what I had to say. I remember nearly passing out over my doctor's desk once, and she still didn't think anything was wrong.

Family members also started questioning my illness and doubting me. I don't blame them to some extent, we look to our doctors for answers, help and trust what they tell us. I remember once rowing with my family, I can't remember what about, I just remember getting so angry. Shouting. Screaming! Why can't they listen, understand and believe me. Crying so hard that I had my first massive panic attack. I couldn't breathe, my heart was thumping, and I was scared, tears streamed down my face. I went dizzy....and I just remember them standing over me saying "look at her! She's gone mad!" and just watching me. I managed to calm myself down, get to bed and I never felt so alone.

With so much physical, emotional and neuro activity constantly going on within us it's no wonder we struggle and feel so ill all the time.

I believe the message of M.E. is about change and acceptance: accept yourself as you are, in this moment, adjust and accept the illness and your limits, listen to what it's trying to tell you. It's not the end. It's a new beginning. A change of lifestyle. A new, calmer lifestyle, slowing you down to see the wonder of the world around you. Yoga is appreciation of life and balance in your world. It may seem far-fetched or you may be having a bad relapse and can't see how or when your life is going to get brighter. Learn to be optimistic. A positive attitude improves our emotional state and healing. Find yourself, find new friends. Start that new hobby you always wanted to do but never found the time to do before. Find the unexpected rewards within this challenging illness. It may be a gateway to a whole new career! It's normal and acceptable to have non-positive days. Cry, sulk, get angry at everything. Release it all, let it all out then take a deep breath and get back on track to finding that path to wellness, health and a happy you.

Recovery from M.E. is very much a long 2 steps forward and 10 steps back road. We rest, feel slightly better, rush to do everything that is needed to be done while we feel up to doing it all and have a burst of energy. Of course, this then results in a relapse and it's back to bed and needing to rest again.

We push ourselves for what? To prove to ourselves we can? To prove to everyone else we aren't lazy? In hope that the illness is over, gone for good and we're back to how we were? Relapses can happen for a number of reasons. Doing too much and pushing ourselves too hard is one. Stress plays a massive part and life will always throw us some type of stress to catch.

Illness on top of illness. Negative and even positive life experiences can drain our bodies of energy. The more you push past the limits of your body, the bigger the relapse can be.

The first important step is to listen to your body. It`s in constant communication with you. Keep a diary of your good times and bad times. They can be up and down day to day or week to week. Finding a pattern will help you plan things and help to avoid a relapse. Learn to know your body's needs, the danger signals, the triggers that make you feel ill and work with them. Look after number one. You! Don`t be afraid to say "no" to anything that could trigger a bad period. By knowing your triggers, you can start to plan lifestyle changes, self-care, diet and work changes to help you balance rest and work. It's a very gradual recovery, pace yourself and when you see the red light flashing. Stop! It`s not worth running that red light.

Don't use energy to fight the illness. I always take Mondays off. It`s my do nothing day. I cope with the weekend, with my daughter and doing things, but Monday as soon as my daughter has gone off to school, it`s me and silence. Rest and re-charge. A day of bed and pjs. Often I get people trying to book me for a Monday, or wanting to come around for a cup of tea. Whereas my head goes yes! You need the money! Or thinks couple of hours will be ok to talk, I know by Wednesday I would be struggling for the rest of the week. My health comes first. It`s used to it. It likes it and is happy with it. I`ve learnt not to feel bad about putting my health first.

Over time, relapses will get less and less severe. They will not last as long and be few and far between. Never, ever lose hope. Stay in this moment, with what you have now and use the time with hobbies and happy future planning. What you do today to help aid recovery sets the path for your future.

Although very few make a total recovery, life can be just as good or even better than it was before getting the illness. It's all to do with your mind-set about the situation and the illness. You can be bitter and angry at it, or you can be grateful for the new opportunities it can and will bring.

I thank it for teaching me. Teaching me patience, gratitude and strength. For getting me into yoga, which is now my full-time job. Without M.E. I wouldn't have been able to learn about yoga, fall in love with practising it and help and see other people benefit from yoga. That makes me happy. I work around my illness. It keeps my aches at bay and my motivation high to do yoga most days. Most importantly it taught me the experiences, stories and lessons which I am now writing in this book to help you. I've seen so many people upset, distraught with the illness and the pain they're suffering. M.E. has broken my heart numerous times over the years. If you believe we all have a life purpose and everything happens for a reason, then I truly believe passing on what I have learnt is mine. I want to help, support and encourage fellow warriors. And I can truly say, I have never been happier than I am now with my life.

You can be too. Listen, write notes and plan your future. It's in your hands. It might not be where you thought you would be. It might not be what you wanted it to be. But you can use the illness to find your sparkle in the world. The world needs you.

List Of Common M.E Symptoms:

This is a general list of symptoms of the illness. There may be more and you may find some don't apply to your condition.

- ✓ Extreme Fatigue / Exhaustion
- ✓ Sleep problems
- ✓ Muscle pain / aches
- ✓ Joint pain
- ✓ Concentration / cognition problems
- ✓ Light / sound sensitivity
- ✓ Body temperature issues.
- ✓ Abdominal pains / bloating
- ✓ Nausea
- ✓ Sinus / nasal issues
- ✓ Swollen glands
- ✓ Sore throat
- ✓ Tender Lymph nodes
- ✓ Headaches
- ✓ Dizziness
- ✓ Weakness
- ✓ Flu symptoms
- ✓ Brain fog
- ✓ Rashes
- ✓ Constant infections
- ✓ Memory loss
- ✓ Slurring speech
- ✓ Muscle spasms
- ✓ Heart problems
- ✓ Irritable Bowel

ॐ About Yoga And How It Can Help You ॐ

We all know yoga has been around for many years, but, have you ever stopped to think why? Maybe, it's because it simply works. It's a complete programme of working body and mind to help heal, focus and strengthen all the systems of the body. The body is controlled by the mind and the mind is controlled by the body. The word yoga means to unite…unite the body and mind to work together in harmony.

You just have to think of some mind-body connections to see this. Think of the most embarrassing moment that has ever happened to you. Yes, the time when THAT happened! Feel the warmth rush to your face and cheeks, you are now blushing aren't you? Now think how you feel when you have a hospital or doctor's appointment, if you see your biggest crush or you are facing your biggest fear. Love, nerves and anxiety bring feelings of butterflies, bats or elephants to the stomach, both examples of mind-body working together just by our thoughts.

Over the years, lots of various forms of yoga have been developed and practised. It's been a "fitness" craze for a lean sculpted body, also yoga dance and cardio yoga. It's been a social media playground for yogis to take selfie pics and show their amazing skills. This can be fine, if that's what you're after from yoga, but it's much more than a daily / weekly workout or selfie snap.

Yoga is not just about the poses, it's actually a way of living, the poses are just a teeny, tiny part of yoga. Originally, poses were practised to help prepare the body and mind before sitting in meditation, while helping to lead the way to a healthier and happier life both on and off the yoga mat.

What I've learnt and what I teach is that yoga is anything you want it to be. It's your flexible friend (pun intended). It's a personal practice. We are all different with different needs, abilities and conditions. Yoga works with your personal goals, wishes, abilities and limitations. Listen to what your body is needing. You don't have to stand on your head, or twist your legs into a pretzel. Your body knows how to heal itself. It will tell you what it needs with warning signs and where you're not 100% right in the body. It will tell you when you need to back away from a pose and where on your body you need a yoga pose, which way to bend and for how long to hold it, to help any aches that you may have. The hardest part is to listen, so you can hear these signs.

The brain and the immune system chat with each other via messages in the nervous system. Illnesses can arise out of a weak immune system, but it's not just outside factors that can weaken the immune system. Mental, emotional and spiritual aspects of your life can also play a big part in sending out positive or negative vibes to your immune system. Yoga can help calm the nervous system, through the poses and breathing. It is about self-awareness and reducing levels of the stress hormone Cortisol, this then calms the nervous system, which in turn calms the body and muscles, resulting in a happier immune system.

Yoga quiets the mind which helps you hear your body and its warning signs better. Just sitting quietly with the sound of the breath, softens the mind, melts tension, worry and anger away. It's quality time between your body and mind. It's quality time for yourself.

Learning to relax to keep our stress levels and anxiety under control can help us deal better with everyday stresses and the illness and gives more clarity. It can reduce mild depression as it helps to increase happy hormones (endorphins) to the brain, our natural feel-good drug.

Yoga postures can help keep joints, muscles, and the lymph system happy. It can help keep the spine supple so that the spine stays strong. Postures also help the body to pump spinal fluid up and down the spine as well as lymph and blood around the body, so that cells are being supplied with the nutrients and oxygen they need for the body to repair itself and to work effectively.

Yoga for M.E. means taking your M.E. symptoms and abilities and working yoga around your M.E, not your M.E. around the yoga. High levels of activity can cause relapses of the illness, yet, not exercising at all can lead to muscle and joints deteriorating and more fatigue. Pace yourself between rest, work and yoga. Slow and steady can achieve long term results.

And finally, yoga can actually give you energy. Who doesn't want a calmer, less stressed, contented body and mind?

List Of Benefits Of Yoga:

- ✓ Maintains muscle strength
- ✓ Releases toxins
- ✓ Adds oxygen to blood and body cells
- ✓ Calms the nervous system
- ✓ Reduces stress
- ✓ Increases mental focus
- ✓ Increases energy
- ✓ Improves digestion
- ✓ Maintains mobility of joints
- ✓ Reduces depression
- ✓ Releases emotions
- ✓ Relieves headaches
- ✓ Relieves muscle aches
- ✓ Massages Lymph system to improve immune system
- ✓ Increases flexibility
- ✓ Encourages body awareness
- ✓ Aids relaxation
- ✓ Relieves anxiety
- ✓ Relieves sleep issues

ॐ Yoga Poses ॐ

There are many benefits of practising the following yoga poses, which for M.E. warriors include: Strengthening the back and spine helping to keep it flexible. Helping posture and preventing bad back issues. Improving breathing, circulation and digestion, keeping the body joints flexible and lubricated. Gently moving the body to help prevent muscle and bone loss. All of which can help greatly if you struggle to move around from day to day. Being bed-ridden with the illness, it`s hard to keep your body nourished and circulation flowing to vital organs for optimum health and recovery.

Yoga helps stretch your whole body, relieving tiredness, tension, aches and tight spots away in body and the mind.

You can go at your pace, do as much or as little as you feel your body needs, whenever it needs it.

Breath during poses should be easy. Back away from the pose if your breathing becomes jerky, if you`re finding it hard to breathe or you find you are holding your breath.

Here's an alphabetical breakdown of all the poses found in this book.

Bridge Pose:

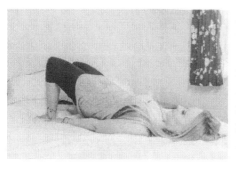

An energy boosting pose, which improves circulation and rejuvenates tired legs and back, stretches the neck and releases neck and chest tension and tension in the spine, hips and the front of the thighs. It strengthens the back, buttocks and hamstrings.

Avoid this pose:

- If you have serious neck or back issues. For mild back pain you may find placing a pillow underneath your tailbone to rest your pelvis on can help.

Lie on the bed and bend your knees, arms beside your body, feet on the bed, hip width apart and bring your heels as close to your buttocks as you comfortably can. Curl your pelvis up towards the ceiling pressing your back to the bed. Hold here if this is enough.

Slowly lift your pelvis, lower back and if you can your middle and upper back off the bed. Raise your hips to the ceiling as you press into the bed with shoulders, arms and feet. Be sure to have an even weight distribution over these points. Lift the chin. Press your shoulder blades against your bed. Breathe deeply for 5 breaths. To come out of the pose, slowly release the spine down to the bed one vertebra at a time.

Camel Pose:

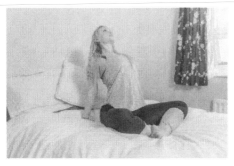

The Camel Pose in this book is a simple modification of the traditional yoga pose. It stretches the entire upper front part of the body, abdominals, chest and throat. It helps improve posture, strengthens the back muscles and stimulates the neck and stomach organs.

Avoid:

- If you suffer from high/low blood pressure
- Migraine
- Insomnia
- Neck injuries

Sitting in Easy Pose, (page 35), place your hands comfortably behind you, fingertips facing the buttocks if you can. Inhale and lift from the chest, arching your back. Tilt your head and neck back if it's comfortable and you have no neck issues. Otherwise keep the neck straight while looking ahead. Move the shoulders down from the ears and squeeze the shoulder blades together. Keep lifting the chest to the ceiling. Keep the belly button drawn into your spine to protect the lower back. Stay and hold here for a few seconds or up to 30 seconds, before slowly straightening up and folding into a gentle Forward Bend over your legs. This helps counteract the pose and the backbend to the spine.

Child`s Pose Extended:

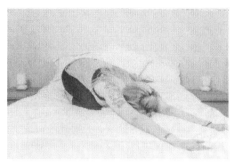

A very relaxing and restorative pose. Helping to relieve stress and tiredness. Reduces anxiety, aids digestion, relieves back pain, and gently stretches ankles, back and hips.

Be cautious:

- If you have knee issues
- High blood pressure

You can go into Child`s Pose between doing any other yoga poses or to rest if you feel the need in the AM yoga chapters. (pages: 52, 55).

Kneel on your bed. Keeping bottom to heels. Stretch forward taking your forehead to the bed. If you wish, you can place a pillow to rest your forehead on. I do this a lot and hug the pillow to relax.

You can either take the arms back along your sides or stretch them out in front of you (as shown) to stretch out the shoulders and release neck tension. Relax all tension from the jaw and facial muscles. Open your shoulders as you breathe. Deep breathe here for 5 full breaths before slowly rounding up to a kneeling position.

Cow Face Pose:

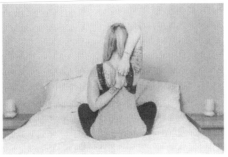 A great chest opener which stretches the shoulders, chest, triceps, armpits and chest. Straightens the spine and helps prevent rounded shoulders, improving posture.

Avoid:

- If you have shoulder and/or neck issues. Try using a strap (dressing gown belt) if your hands don't reach to clasp. Keep your head and gaze straight in front of you.

Sit in Easy Pose (page 35), keeping your back straight. Lengthen up from the waist. Raise your right hand up and back over your right shoulder so that it sits between your shoulder blades. Take your left arm and move it around the left side, bringing it up to clasp the right hand. Don't worry if you can't reach. With practice and learning to release muscle tension the clasp will happen in time. Keep lengthening up while holding the stretch. Hold for up to 30 seconds. Repeat on the left side.

Easy Pose:

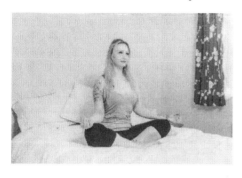

A great relaxing pose to begin your yoga practice, breathing work and meditation. Stretches the hips, knees and ankles. Strengthens the back, stimulates pelvis and spine. Calms mind and body

Sit comfortably on your bed. Spine straight without strain and avoid rounding the shoulders. You can sit back against the headboard or wall to help balance and keep the spine straight. Place your feet so they`re in line, one in front of the other and heels as close to the hips as is comfortable for you. If you have tight hamstrings, lower back, or hips another method is to cross your shins to find even balance in the hips. For any knee or ankle issues, you can place pillows under your knees to support them. Keep lifting up from the waist, chest and head to create space for the breath to flow around your body with ease. Place hands on your knees or for breath work you can place hands on your abdominals. Stay in this pose for as long as you wish.

Easy Pose Cat And Cow Stretch:

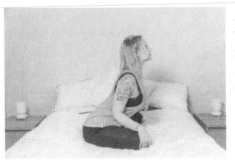

A modified yoga pose which helps to stretch neck and spine. Strengthens abdominals.

Avoid:

- Neck movement if you suffer from neck issues.

Follow the guide to sit comfortably into Easy Pose. Place your hands onto your knees. Relax your shoulders and lift the chest and the top of your head to the ceiling. On an inhale, arch your back, look up being careful not to compress your neck and take the shoulders down the back. Press hands into your knees for support.

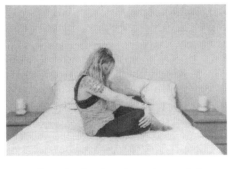

On an exhale, round your spine, take your chin to the chest and straighten your arms, keeping hands on your knees to stretch out the shoulder blades. Inhale, arch the back again and exhale rounding the back. Flow through however many rounds of this pose you need. Work with the breath as your guide.

Easy Pose Neck Rolls:

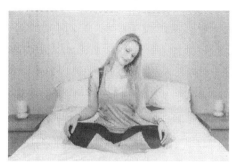 A simple yoga pose to relieve tension from the neck and shoulders. Stretches the neck joints and relieves stiffness. Helps to bring circulation to the face and head.

Avoid:

- If you suffer serious neck issues
- Headaches

Follow the guide to sit comfortably into Easy Pose. Place your hands onto your knees. Relax your shoulders and lift the chest and the top of your head to the ceiling. Slowly take your right ear to your right shoulder. Draw the shoulders down the back so you feel the tension release from the left side of the neck. Hold for 5 breaths before slowly rolling the chin down to your chest, hold for 5 breaths. Don't force the chin to the chest just let it comfortably hang there. Slowly roll the head to the left, so that your left ear is down to your left shoulder. Draw the shoulders down the back so you feel the stretch along the right side of your neck. Hold for 5 breaths. Repeat: this time from left to right

Easy Pose Side Bends:

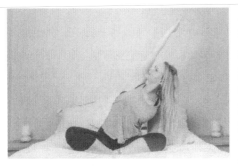

A stretch to open up the rib cage, waist and hip. Stretches your hips, knees and ankles. Strengthens your back. Stimulates pelvis and spine. Stretches shoulders, chest and sides of the body. Calms mind and body.

Follow the guide for Easy Pose. After a few deep steady breaths inhale and raise both arms up above the head in prayer position. Palms touching if you can. On the exhale take the left arm down to the left side a foot or so away from the left hip. Keeping the left ear away from the left shoulder, lean over to the left. Keeping the right arm extended over the right ear. Feel the stretch along the right side of the neck, shoulder and right rib cage to waist. Try to keep the right hip down on the bed, and shoulders away from the ears. Hold the pose for 5 breaths before inhaling to the centre and then exhaling down to the right side.

Easy Pose Twist:

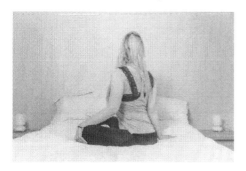 A gentle spinal twist to detox organs and bring blood flow to the spinal column. Stretches your hips, knees and ankles. Strengthens your back. Stimulates pelvis and spine.

Detoxifies the digestive system. Calms mind and body.

Avoid:

- If you suffer from IBS flare up
- High/low blood pressure
- Insomnia
- Headache

Follow the guide for Easy Pose. Take a few slow deep breaths to clear your mind and relax your body. When you are ready, on an inhale lift from the waist feeling the crown of the head lift to the ceiling. Take the shoulders down the back. On the exhale, twist from the waist to your left. Keeping the hips square to the front as you can. Place your left hand behind you and right hand on the inside of the right knee. Stay here for 5 breaths and then on an exhale twist again from the shoulders keeping the head lifted and upright and slowly turn to look over your left shoulder if you have no neck issues. Take a few deep breaths before exhaling back to the centre. Take a deep inhale and on the exhale repeat to the right side.

Half Locust Pose:

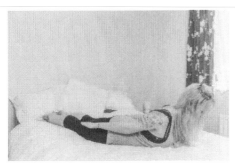 A backbend which helps energize the body. Fights fatigue. Reduces stress and improves the posture which helps with breathing issues.

It also tones the back and reduces mild lower back pain. Tones the buttocks and hamstrings. Stretches the shoulders, chest, abdominals and thighs.

Avoid:

- If you suffer with headaches
- Have serious back and / or neck issues

You can keep forehead to the bed or on a pillow for neck support. And just raise your arms, taking the shoulder blades and arms away from your ears.

Lie face down on your bed. Place a pillow or folded blanket under your forehead to support the neck. Place your arms alongside your body, palms down. Point your toes. Inhale and press the feet into the bed as you raise the head, shoulders and chest off the bed. Keep belly button drawn into your spine. Breathe slowly and deeply and hold the pose for 5-10 seconds before lowering it down on an exhale.

Knees To Chest Pose:

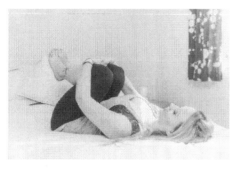

A calming, comforting and a gentle massage to the body and mind. Massages the back and abdominal organs. Stretches the lower back, hip flexors and buttocks. Relieves mild menstrual pains. Aids digestion.

Avoid:

- If you suffer from stomach upsets
- Heavy menstrual cycle
- High blood pressure
- Slipped disc
- Neck, knee, spine or hip injuries

Lie on your bed. Legs straight down in front of you. On an inhale, slowly bend the knees and bring knees to chest. Legs together. If you find this too much, you can raise one knee at a time. Keeping the opposite leg down on the bed. On an exhale, hug the knees into your chest with your arms. You can stay still here, or you can rock the legs from side to side. Or take the knees into slow circles to release the hips. If you want to further the pose, inhale and on the exhale, lift your head and chest off the bed and bring your forehead to your knees. Press the knees to the chest and your back into the bed. Inhale, lift the head away from the knees and exhale taking the head and your legs back down onto the bed to rest.

Legs In The Air:

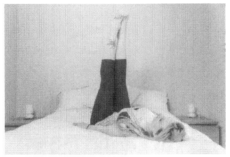

You can do this on your bed with your legs up against the headboard or a wall for a relaxing, restorative pose.

Eases anxiety, premenstrual cramps. Relieves tired legs and lower back pain. Stretches hamstrings, lower back and legs.

Avoid:

- If you are menstruating
- Pregnant
- Have high blood pressure
- Glaucoma

Take the pillows away and shift your bottom as close to the headboard as possible. Slowly bring the legs up to rest on the wall or headboard. Keep the legs as straight as possible to stretch the backs of the legs for a few breaths, before letting the legs naturally fall open, relax your knees and feet and relax into the pose. You can incorporate foot rolls or point and flex the feet to relax and keep the ankle and foot joints supple.

One-Legged Forward Fold:

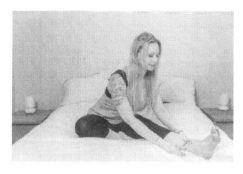 A gentle stress relieving, calming forward fold, which can help relieve mild depression, and lower back pain. Stretches hamstrings, groin, spine and shoulders. While massaging the abdominal organs.

Avoid:

- If you suffering from asthma
- IBS flare up
- Knee injuries

Sit on your bed with both legs out straight in front of you. Keep your back straight and chest lifted so you're not rounding the spine. Take your right leg and bend it so that the right foot touches the inside of your left thigh. If you have tight hips or knees you can place a pillow under the right knee to support it. Inhale and raise your arms, lifting the chest. On the exhale, fold from the hips and (not your back) down over the straight left leg. Think about lengthening down and not rounding down to the leg. You can use a dressing gown belt to hook over the left foot and hold with your hands to help keep your spine straight. Keep the left knee soft and slightly bent to avoid injury. Breathe deeply and slowly. Stay in the pose for as long as you want. Come back to sitting on an inhale and repeat on the other leg.

Reclining Spinal Twist:

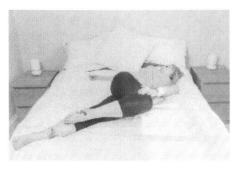

A detoxing twist to spine and organs. Helps stimulate circulation. increases spinal flexibility. Stretches spine. Eliminates toxins from the body. Aids digestion.

Caution:

- Lower back issues

Lie on your back on your bed. Take your arms out to either side shoulder height, palms down. Bend your right leg, keeping your legs together. On an exhale, slowly take your knee down over to the left side. Placing your right foot onto your left shin. If you have no neck issues, you can then exhale and slowly look over to your right hand. This gives a full spinal stretch and twist to stimulate the spinal nerves and helps spinal fluid to flow easily. Stay for 5 breaths. On an inhale slowly raise back to the centre. Take a couple of breaths here before on an exhale taking the left knee to the right side and looking over to your left hand. Stay for 5 breaths before returning to centre.

Savasana:

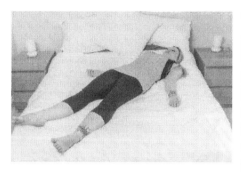

The easiest looking pose to the eye. The hardest pose to master. "Really!?" I hear you say. How can just lying there be that hard? The easiest way to explain is this: think of all the times you wanted to sleep. Hours tick by and your body is fidgeting or your mind is on a whirlwind of problems which you can't switch off. The purpose of Savasana is to try and completely relax both body and mind to a still state. Like when you're meditating

This pose is the most rewarding for M.E. warriors as it helps recharge your batteries and clears any stress and exhaustion from the body and mind. It invigorates and refreshes, yet the smooth deep breathing soothes the nerves and quietens the mind.

Lie down on your bed, under the covers so that you are nice and warm and muscles stay relaxed. Let the legs naturally fall apart. Place a rolled up blanket underneath your knees if you have lower back issues, keep arms either by your side, palms up or place them on your stomach. Move your shoulders down away from your ears. Relax your face and jaw. If you find that your face or any area of your body tenses up during this pose, (shoulders, back and jaw being the most common stress holders of the body), take a deep breath in and on the exhale, consciously relax that area. Close your eyes and start to focus on your breath. Breathe slowly and deeply. You can focus on the rise and fall of your stomach. You can count or use a mantra to help calm your mind. Feel your body getting heavier as it relaxes. Feel it slowly start to sink into the bed. Feel yourself safe, comfortable and stress free.

You can do this pose on its own, before calmly drifting off to a happy sleep at night.

Seated Forward Bend:

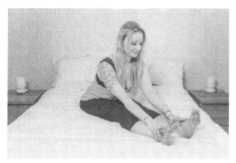

A lovely pose which reduces stress and calms the mind and body. Stretches spine, shoulders, hamstrings. Helps relieve mild depression. Improves the digestive system.

Benefits the nervous system.

Caution:

- Hamstring issues
- Lower back issues
- If you are an asthma sufferer

Sit on your bed, legs outstretched in front of you. Place a pillow under your buttocks if you need to for support if your hips and hamstrings are tight. Keep the toes flexed (toes pointing towards you) and ankles as close together as you can. Keeping your chest lifted and spine comfortably upright, on an inhale, lift up from the waist raising your arms, on an exhale, slowly fold forward, bending from the hips and not the chest or waist (don't round the spine). Go as far as your body allows, don't push. You're aiming to move the chest to the knees not your head, focus on lengthening down to the legs and not the depth of the pose. You can use a dressing gown strap placed around the balls of the feet to hold, which helps keep your alignment. Breathe as you relax into the pose, stay as long as possible to release tight muscles and tension. On an inhale slowly raise back up.

Stretch Pose:

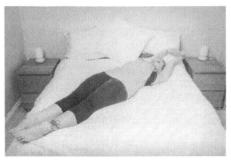

Not really a yoga pose, but who doesn't like to stretch? We all love a great big stretch in the morning or as we get into bed at night so I've included it in this book. After you have finished your yoga, before you settle down to meditate or sleep, a few big stretches will do wonders for your body and mind.

While in Savasana, inhale and take your arms up and over your head. Exhale. Then on an inhale stretch your arms away from your head as far as you can, spread your fingers wide. Flex your wrists and at the same time stretch your feet away from your legs as far as you can. Point or flex the feet or do both. Arch your back, sway (think of how a cat stretches in the sun). There's no right or wrong way to do this. Take a moment to feel where on your body you need to hold a stretch, or which way your body wants to go and do that. The only DO with this pose would be, to do it with a smile on your face.

Through The Needle Pose:

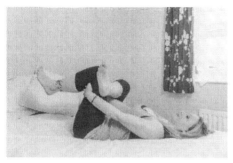 A relaxing but strong pose to help relieve stress and anxiety from the mind. It helps to stretch the hip muscles. Lengthens lower back. Tones the quads and hamstrings. Improves circulation in the lower body and can reduce pain that is caused by inactivity. It can also reduce digestive and menstrual pain.

Avoid:

- Serious hip or knee issues

From lying on your back. Bend your knees so your feet are flat on the bed, hip width apart. Take your right foot and place it on top of your left thigh. Keep right foot flexed. Inhale and on an exhale bring the legs towards your chest. If you can, take your hands and place them around your left thigh. If this is too much, you can use a dressing gown strap. Make sure your shoulders are away from the ears. Hold for as long as comfortable. Release the left leg back down on the bed on an exhale. Repeat on the other leg.

Wide Angle Seated Forward Bend:

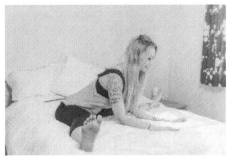 A restorative pose which reduces stress and calms the mind. Stretches spine, shoulders, inner thighs, hamstrings. Helps relieve mild depression and anxiety. Improves digestion. Benefits the nervous system.

Cautious:

- Hamstring issues
- Lower back issues
- If you are an asthma sufferer

Sit on your bed, stretch your legs wide and straight to either side of the bed. You can place a pillow under your buttocks if you need to for support if your hips and hamstrings are tight. Keep the toes flexed (toes pointing towards you). Keep the chest lifted and spine comfortably upright. On an inhale, lift up from the waist raising your arms. On an exhale, slowly fold forward, bending from the hips and not the chest or waist (don't round the spine). Go as far as your body allows, don't push. You're aiming the chest towards the bed not your head. Place hands in front of you on the bed. Breathe as you relax into the pose, stay as long as possible to release tight muscles and tension. On an inhale slowly raise back up.

ॐ Yoga Sequences ॐ

Sometimes we all get too tired to do anything. I do try to pick one pose which I know would help me that day. Whether it be a gentle backbend to fill me with some positive energy or a forward bend to help me relax. There is always something that yoga can bring to your day. It doesn't matter if you do 1 or 100 poses. Make yoga YOUR yoga.

The following sequences don't have any "rules" as we all feel different day to day. So follow the sequences or hold the pose/s as you wish. Breathe into the poses. If you struggle - back away. If they feel great, hold for as long as you want. Don't just hold the poses. Breathe them. Feel and scan your body while in a pose to see how it is feeling. I find the ones I struggle with (not a painful struggle) are the poses I most need. So I try to hold these a little longer.

Notice throughout, if you are tensing muscles in your body or face. Tensing muscles will prevent you from doing the pose, enjoying the pose and holding it with ease. It will also use up body energy. Relax the muscles. Let gravity take you into the poses rather than forcing your body into them.

ॐ Yoga Sequence AM 5 Minutes ॐ

Awaken your body with this 5-minute yoga sequence to stretch your spine and joints.

Follow the instructions on previous pages for each pose: Full Body Stretch: page 48, Easy Pose: page 35, Easy Pose Twist: page 39, Easy Pose Side Bends: page 38, Cow Face Pose: page 34, Easy Pose Camel: page 32, Seated Forward Bend: page 47.

Hold the poses as is right for you (recommended time is added). Repeat the sequence twice if you wish.

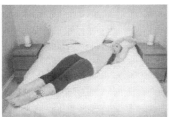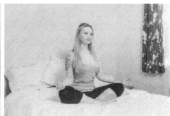

Begin with 4 Full Body Stretches to awaken body and mind, before slowly coming up to sit in Easy Pose, take 5 deep full breaths here.

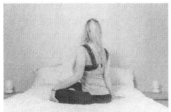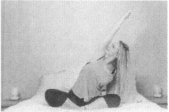

On an inhale. Raise the arms and come into Easy Pose Twist to your right. Hold for 5 breaths. Return to centre before twisting to the left. Hold for 5 breaths and return to centre.

Inhale. Take arms back up above your head and come into Easy Pose Side Bends. Take 5 breaths to each side. Come to centre and take a few deep breaths.

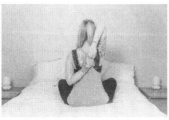 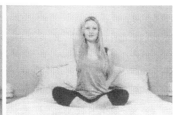

On an inhale. Take your right arm up and over into Cow Face Pose. Clasp if you can (or use a strap). Breathe for 5 full breaths. Repeat on the left side. Come back to Easy Pose and relax for a minute.

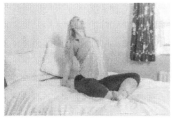 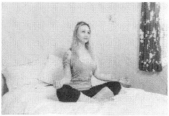

Then taking your hands behind you place them on the bed. Come into Easy Pose Camel, stay for 5 breaths, before exhaling back into Easy Pose.

Stretch out both your legs in front of you. Come into Seated Forward Bend. Stay here for 5 breaths.

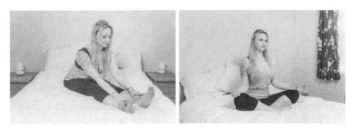

Slowly roll up your upper body and come back into Easy Pose. Take 5 full breaths here and note how your body is feeling.

ॐ Yoga Sequence AM 10 Minutes ॐ

If you have a little longer in the mornings or just want to add to your yoga practice to help you through the day follow the sequence below for an all over wake-up body yoga practice. Again hold the poses as your body needs (up to 5 deep breaths if you can).

Full Body Stretch: page 48, Easy Pose: page 35, Easy Pose Twist: page 39, Easy Pose Side Bend: page 38, Cow Face Pose: page 34, Easy Pose Camel: page 32, Half Locust Pose: page 40, Bridge Pose: page 31, One-Legged Fold: page 43, Easy pose Cat/cow: page 36.

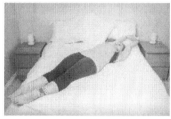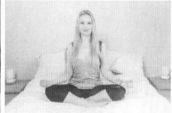

Begin taking 4 Full Body Stretches to waken body and mind before coming to sitting in Easy Pose for 5 full breaths.

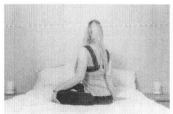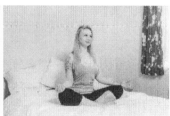

Inhale and take the arms up over your head into Prayer Pose if you can. On the exhale, twist from your lower abdominals over to your right side, Easy Pose Twist. Stay for 5 breaths. Twisting more with each exhale. Inhale come to centre. Exhale twist to the left for 5 breaths.

Return to Easy Pose. Inhale and exhale into Easy Pose Side Bends, taking 5 breaths to each side. Come back to Easy Pose.

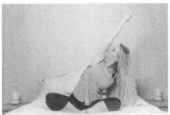 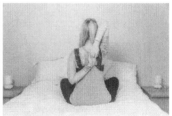

When you are ready, inhale and take your right arm up and over your shoulder coming into Cow Face Pose, stay here for 5 breaths and release to change to the left side. Hold for 5 breaths and relax into Easy Pose for a moment.

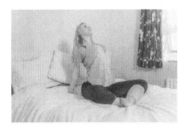

Take your hands behind your back and onto the bed. Come into Camel Pose. Stretch the whole upper body for 5 breaths before coming into an Easy Forward Bend to counteract the back bending for 5 breaths.

Come to lying on your front. Take a moment to settle and get comfortable. When you are ready, breathe into Half Locust Pose. It's a challenging pose and you often find yourself holding your breath! Breathe and slowly build up the breaths in your own time. (5 breaths eventually). Relax and return to lying on your back. Take a moment to ground your body into the bed. Take your time.

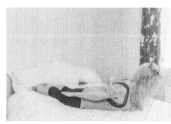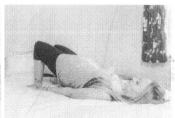

Slowly come into Bridge Pose. Try to hold for 5 breaths. Again slowly build up strength and breaths in your own time. Relax before coming up to Easy Pose.

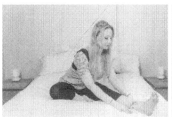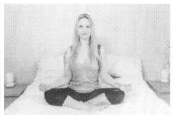

Taking your legs out straight in front of you. Come into One-Legged Fold. Remembering to keep spine long. Take 5 deep breaths here. Then switch legs for 5 breaths before sitting back into Easy Pose.

From here, place your hands on your knees and come into Easy Pose Cat/Cow Pose. Flowing with your breath. Inhale and look up, exhale, round and stretch. Repeat up to 10 times.

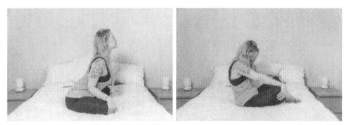

Then come to sit in Easy Pose. Close your eyes and note how your body and mind are feeling before you start your day

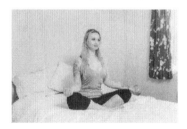

ॐ PM 5 Minute Relax Yoga ॐ

A simple, gentle and relaxing sequence to release aches in lower back and calm the nervous system before sleep. Follow the instructions for each pose on the previous pages and hold the poses for up to 10 breaths.

Easy Pose: page 35, Easy Pose Neck Rolls: page 37, Easy Pose Side Bends: page 38, Child`s Pose Extended: page 33, Knees To Chest Pose: page 41, Reclining Spinal Twist: page 44, Full Body Stretch: page 48, Savasana: page 45.

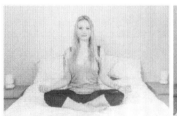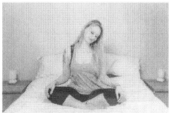

Come to sitting on your bed in Easy Pose. Close your eyes and focus on your breath. Start by slowing your breath down and taking 10 deep full breaths.

When you`re ready, begin by doing Easy Pose Neck Rolls 4 times each side. Work with your breath. If your neck and shoulders are particularly tight, you may like to hold the stretch each side for a couple of breaths too. Come back to the centre slowly.

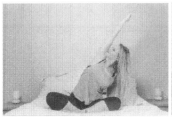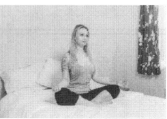

Take a deep inhale and raise your arms up over your head into prayer pose (if you can). On an exhale take your right arm onto the bed and your left arm up over your body. Come into Easy Side Stretch Pose. Stay here for 10 breaths. Slowly come back to centre on an inhale. Exhale and take your left arm to the bed and your right arm up and over your body. Stay for 10 breaths before returning to Easy Pose.

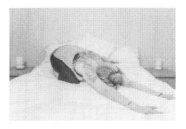

Take a moment to relax and notice how you feel. Come onto all fours on your bed and come into Child`s Pose Extended. Stretch out the arms in front of you to release upper back tension. Focus on 10 deep breaths in this pose before slowly rolling up to a kneeling position.

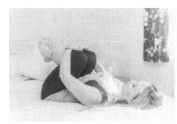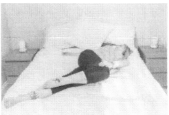

Come to lying on your back. Take a moment to settle into the bed. Come into Knees to Chest pose. Close your eyes and breathe, if you wish to relieve lower back pain or premenstrual cramps, rock or move side to side as you carry out 10 breaths.

On an exhale, straighten the legs out in front of you and come into Reclining Spinal Twists, taking 10 breaths to each side.

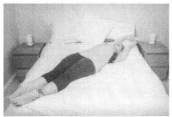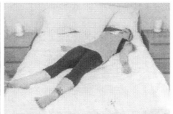

Taking your legs back out in front of you on the bed. Inhale and raise your arms up over your head. Take 5 big Full Body Stretches feeling every muscle start to relax.

From this come gently into Savasana. Feel free to get under the duvet or a blanket before resting in Savasana to stay warm as you gently drift off to sleep

ॐ PM 10 Minute Relax Yoga ॐ

For a longer relaxation, releasing aches and tension from the body follow the suggested sequence below. Breathe deeply for 10 full breaths and feel the tension wash away. Wrap yourself under your blanket before the final pose to help you drift off to sleep.

Easy Pose: page 35, Easy Pose Neck Rolls: page 37, Easy Pose Cat/Cow: page 36, Child's pose: page 33, Wide Angle Seated Bend: page 50, Knees To Chest Pose: page 41, Through The Needle Pose: page 49, Legs In The Air Pose: page 42, Reclining Spinal Twist: page 44, Savasana: page 45.

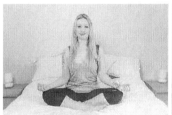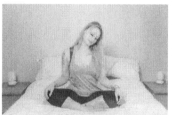

Begin by sitting comfortably in Easy Pose. Gently take your attention to your breath as you slowly start to deepen and lengthen the breath with Full Body Breathing (page 76). Stay here with your eyes closed for 10 breaths. Let go of the day.

When you're ready. Come into Easy Pose Neck Rolls. Work with your breath to flow side to side, 5 times each side. Hold the pose if you have tension in the neck. Come back to centre in Easy Pose.

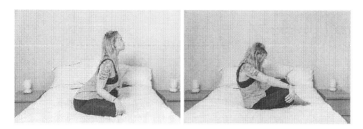

From Easy Pose, move into Cat/Cow Pose. Flowing with your breath, inhale looking up and arching your spine, exhale and round the spine, taking chin to chest. Repeat for 10 breaths.

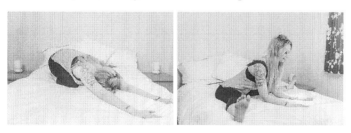

Then come to all fours on your bed and move into Child`s Pose. Take 10 long deep breaths here. Feel the tension wash away from your face. Come up from Child`s Pose and stretch your legs out and wide in front of you, coming into Wide Angle Seated Bend. Place your hands in front of you on the bed. Keep the spine long and fold forward at the hips. Keep the knees soft. Stay here for 10 breaths. As you relax, you will find you get a little further into this pose with every exhale. Come up on an inhale and move to lie on your back. Settle into the bed.

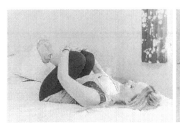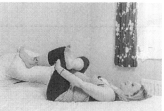

When you`re ready, bring your knees into your chest. Close your eyes and stay here for 10 breaths. Rock or move knees side to side to release the lower back if you wish. Release the arms and take your feet to the bed hip width apart.

Inhale and place your left foot over onto your right thigh. Take your arms through to hold onto the right leg. Exhale and bring the right leg towards your chest. Keep the right knee bent Through the Needle Pose. Stay here for 10 breaths. Releasing the hips, on an exhale lower the legs. Inhale and switch sides for 10 breaths. Exhale and release legs.

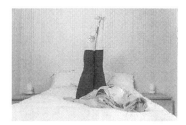

Bring both legs extended up straight into Legs In The Air Pose (you can do this against a headboard or a wall). Close your eyes and stay here for as long as you wish, focusing on your gentle breathing.

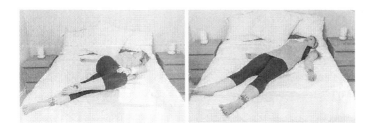

When you are ready. Slowly release legs down from the air (or wall/headboard) and come to lie on your back. Inhale and take your right foot to left shin, bending the knee. On an exhale, take the right knee over to the left side, Reclining Spinal Twist Pose. Hold for 10 breaths. Inhale come to centre. Exhale release the leg. Switch sides and hold for 10 breaths. Inhale return to centre.

Exhale and come into Savasana. Close your eyes. Let your breathing be calm and normal. Follow with a meditation or simply just stay here until you naturally drift off to sleep.

ॐ Quick Pick Me Up Yoga ॐ

All too often we have our times where we need a quick pick me up to get through the rest of the day. We reach for the caffeine or sugar for a quick fix. Next time, try one or all of these energy boosting poses to wake up mind and muscles for a little bit of get-up-and-go.

Easy Pose Cat: page 36, Half Locust Pose: page 40, Cow Face Pose: page 34, Easy Pose Side Bends: page 38.

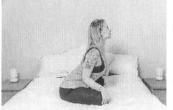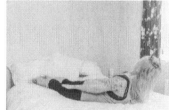

Easy Pose Cat Pose helps wake up and loosen the spine, which is perfect if you have been sitting or lying for long periods of time. Half Locust Pose, stimulates the abdominal organs, releases shoulder and neck tension and improves breathing. Great pose if you have been slouching over a desk or awkwardly lying on the sofa for a while.

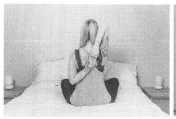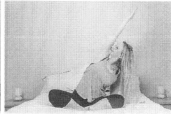

Cow Face Pose is great again if you have been driving or sat at a desk. It helps release neck and shoulder tension which can help prevent tension headaches. Easy Pose Side Bends help wake up the body. Boosting and helping circulation flow better throughout your body while releasing stiffness in the upper body, which can lead to a slouching posture and aches in the body.

If you feel yourself and your body getting tired and aching, pick and carry out the pose or poses that will help your body. It can vary from day to day. Some days you may want to do all the poses. Some days just one and repeat it a few times. There are no rules with yoga. Listen to your body. Pick a pose. Carry it out according to your body`s need. Repeat. It`s that simple.

Yoga can be adapted to everyone`s individual needs and abilities.

ॐ Yoga For A Bad Day ॐ

Sometimes M.E. takes all our energy. We can't sit up or move very much. Lying and resting is all we can manage. Below is a simple flare-up yoga pose / sequence you can do on a bad day to help keep oxygen and circulation flowing through your body, helping to heal your body. Hold and breathe each pose for a few minutes, repeat as many times as you wish during the day or night.

I'm not putting any time for these poses. On bad days I can range from holding poses for just 3 breaths to 3 minutes. So, follow your body's needs.

Full Body Stretch: page 48, Reclining Spinal Twist: page 44, Knees To Chest: page 41, Savasana: page 45.

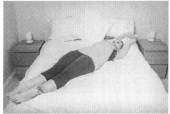 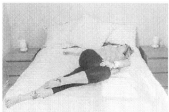

Full Body Stretch and Reclining Spinal Twist.

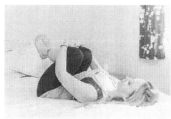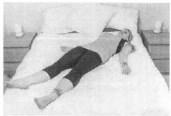

Knees To Chest and Savasana.

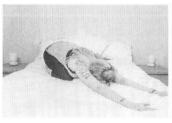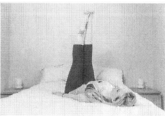

Child`s Pose and Legs In The Air Pose.

Breathe and take time to relax.

Remember bad days will happen. Don't be too hard on yourself and don't feel guilty for taking time out to rest, sleep and stretch out. Mindset is everything. Try to read or watch funny films. Keeping your spirits up boosts happy hormones helping bad days to not seem so bad or last very long. Laughter is the best medicine so they say.

ॐ Breathe Easy & Meditate ॐ

I didn't start getting into meditation until very recently. It goes hand in hand with yoga but my body and mind just weren't ready for the meditation side.

I could sit for hours doing nothing for sure, but meditation was something else. I would get restless and bored. I would check my phone. I would have an itch. "Am I allowed to scratch it? Have I sat for 5 minutes?" "Whoop! I did it…nope I didn't. It was only 1 minute and 12 seconds, yikes! Doesn't time drag! I need a cuppa and will try again tonight".

I tried on and off to empty my mind. I really tried forcing emptiness and darkness behind my eyelids, the more I tried, the more energy I was using up and the more thoughts swarmed into my head. A busy mind is exhausting!

Looking back, the problem was I was trying TOO hard. I thought I had to literally empty and stop every thought popping into my head. I would give up as soon as the first thought popped up thinking I had failed.

Stilling both body and mind is a skill. It's hard to do, but can be done and has been done. I have finally learnt that thoughts will always pop up, I can't stop them it's what they do. I just have to smile and let them be there like clouds in the sky. Just see them but not react to them until I've finished and then I can go about my day.

It's again trial and error with meditation. I found it's very personal and a technique that works for me may not work for someone else. I actually love sitting there and meditating now. I've slowly built up time gradually. The best way is to practise, little and often and don't get frustrated or give up. I feel re-newed, have more energy inside me afterwards, and come away with a smile and feel positive about whatever I was meditating on that day. I now try to meditate twice a day although sometimes it`s not possible, but I do try to squeeze in some me time even if it`s just for 5 or 10 minutes, especially if I feel a surge of tiredness creeping up. I set the timer on my phone and "just be" until it pings time`s up. 20 minutes of deep relaxation can be more beneficial to the energy levels than 5 hours` sleep.

For M.E. sufferers, relaxation is one of the most needed aspects for recovery, but it`s also the hardest thing to do with all the struggles we face day to day. Feeling weak and ill and having to cope with everyday stresses, we need energy to help heal our bodies, but our bodies are out of energy.

Relaxation and meditation can boost energy levels and have a great healing effect on both body and mind. They can help the mind and body to rest deeply. While calming the nervous system, they heal and balance the immune system. They can help prevent panic and anxiety attacks, help free muscle tension in the body, and help balance our emotional state of being, so we can cope with everyday stress a lot easier.

Exhaustion is your body`s way of telling you to stop! It has had enough and isn't doing any more until it`s rested. Don't fight your body. Don't try to push it. Your body knows how to heal itself, so for your health, give it what it wants. A rest.

You can meditate morning, noon or night. I find I start to flag during the afternoon around 5 or 6pm. I use this time to switch off from the world to sit and relax. You can start with just 5 minutes and build up. If your body is needing more than 20 minutes add more. Go with your flow. Use this time for positive vibes to enter your body, mind and soul.

Alone time re-charges your batteries and helps you clear your mind. It helps you focus on what really matters. YOU. Your healing, your needs, your goals, YOU! Your life, your dreams, your wishes. Use this time to befriend the one that will always be by your side. YOU. Find yourself, be optimistic, dream your recovery, and start to believe in YOU. And if at any time you start to doubt yourself you can go to that alone place where your friend is, she / he will help you see that you're not alone, you are strong, and you can do this.

It all starts with proper breathing. We breathe in and out every second of every day without even thinking about it. We take it for granted until there's a problem which makes us aware of it. Most of the time we are unaware that we are actually breathing incorrectly day to day.

Our body is our energy system. We need to heal our body and healing needs energy. Our cells depend on oxygen and energy to help heal us and we can work on building energy in the body by the use of deep breathing techniques and improving our breath on a daily basis.

Correct breathing, not only keeps the lungs healthy, our heart, brain and blood get maximum oxygen as well to help heal. It also releases emotional tension in the mind and muscle tension from the body.

Most of us breathe from the chest, maybe expanding the ribs too. Our lungs aren't being used to their full capacity and our bodies are oxygen deprived. Shallow breathing can make anxiety and panic attacks worse, can cause headaches from lack of oxygen flowing to the brain and cause tense shoulders and neck. It can also LOWER energy levels.

If you only have 3 minutes to spare in your day, use those precious seconds to tune in to your breath with Full Body Breath (page 76). Be aware of your stomach. Breathe in and expand the tummy out, like a balloon. Feel the air fill upwards to ribs, lungs and chest. Then slowly exhale, feeling the air fall from the chest, ribs and stomach drawing in towards the spine. Repeat.

Benefits of Meditation:

- ✓ Calms the mind and aids relaxation
- ✓ Gives the brain and body more energy
- ✓ Relieves anxiety
- ✓ Relieves insomnia
- ✓ Helps you to manage emotions
- ✓ Helps aid concentration
- ✓ Lowers blood pressure
- ✓ Decreases muscle tension
- ✓ Improves breathing
- ✓ Lowers stress levels
- ✓ Aids better sleep
- ✓ Builds self-confidence

ॐ Start Meditating ॐ

Find the right place for you. Make it cozy, warm and comfortable. If it`s summer, I love sitting in the sun with the breeze on my face. If it`s winter, I sit by a heater with fairy lights and candles around me. I also meditate when lying in bed morning, afternoon or before sleep. You can try playing soothing music but I find silence really is golden for this. Switch phones off. Avoid the world and people for the set time. This is YOUR time.

Wear comfortable clothes (or pjs). Stretch the body (page 48) a few times before settling down to meditate. This prevents muscle stiffness and fidgeting.

Start small. Set a timer for 5 minutes at first and slowly after a few weeks build it up to 10 minutes, then 15 etc.

There are lots of different methods to help you focus, to help meditation and to calm you. Try different methods to find one that's suitable for you and that you enjoy.

Place hands on your tummy to feel the breath. Close eyes and visualize. Light a candle or have a picture close by to focus your gaze upon.

Don't give up! It takes time and 1 minute is still more beneficial to you than none.

ॐ My Everyday Meditation ॐ

I'm going to talk you through my own meditation routine with added options. If you find my way doesn't work for you, then change things to suit your personal likes, your space and how you are feeling.

Start by focusing on your breathing. How are you breathing? Are you breathing from your chest? Breath can affect your health and emotions so take your attention to your stomach. You can place your hands on your stomach to help you focus while carrying out Full Body Breathing Technique below.

While breathing in and out through your nose, inhale slowly and expand the tummy, carry the inhale up to your ribs and feel them expand outwards creating space. Carry the inhale to the chest feeling the sternum lift upwards. Smile! Then on the exhale work down. Let the chest relax, let the rib cage contract and let the stomach draw into the spine to remove every last bit of air. Don't rush, the slower the better. Repeat as many times as you want or feel the need. The first few times I did this I got light headed so please go gently. It's your body and brain getting used to the massive amount of oxygen and it should pass after a few days.

Conscious breathing helps you to become more aware of how to breathe, your awareness can then be used to help you feel calm under stress or panic. It refreshes the mind and boosts your concentration. It also lowers blood pressure and relieves tension. It can also help promote a deeper sleep.

Once you have steadied your breathing for a few moments you have a choice. Either stay focusing on your stomach if that's working for you. Sometimes that's all that's needed. Sometimes you need different things from the meditation to help your mind on the more challenging days.

For bad days where my mind can't get calm or I feel an emotional wreck, I pick a mantra or an intention to keep repeating in my head throughout the meditation time. I found it easier to start with repeating just one mantra. It gave my mind something to "play" with for the duration of the relaxation period. How you think is important. Thinking and thoughts are energy. Negative thoughts and thinking can drain and tire you. Positive thoughts can uplift and brighten your mood.

I always start with 10 deep slow inhales and exhales, to relax then I add the mantra. Mantras can be anything to help you with how you are at that moment.

My day to day favourite mantra is: "Everything is fine". Think of the words flowing as you breathe in and out. Repeat for the duration of the meditation. Other great mantras are: inhale… "Faith", exhale…. "Fear". Say this repeatedly in your mind for a while. Feel your breath, as your mind and body start to relax.

If you want, add more positive affirmations such as:

"I am healthy". "I am getting better every day". "Happy and healthy". "Everything is going to be ok". "I am strong". "Life is great".

The mantras can be anything that is personal to you. I find I change mine depending on how I feel. Repeat them, believe them and then repeat them some more.

These mantras will help keep your mind focused on something, so you can relax and heal.

If you find yourself thinking "my ass is numb" or "surely it`s been 5 minutes!" Don`t judge yourself, don't get frustrated. Let the thought pass. Take a deep inhale and just keep repeating your magical words. Focus on those until the timer says "well done" you did it.

ॐ Meditation For Stress ॐ

Sometimes things happen in a blink of an eye and cause us instant stress, making us panic and worry in a split second. An appointment, results, family issues or bad news are just a few things we sometimes can`t plan. This is what I personally do in those "stress hits me in the face, what am I going to do?!" moments. Everyone is different and it obviously depends on the type of stress that's happening.

I shut myself away. Not for long, 30 mins - maximum. If that's not possible, excuse yourself if you are with people to go to the bathroom. Sit and breathe for a few minutes. Breathe. Deep, slow breaths that calm your mind and heart-rate. Listen to your body, your emotions. Are your muscles tight? Do you feel teary? Weak? Shaky? How high on a stress scale are you feeling? Be aware of how you think. Don't over-think or analyze your thoughts or the stress just check in, acknowledge them and carry on focusing on your deep breathing. I mantra a lot. Not out loud. Just repeating a short sentence over and over in my head until I feel calmer. This could be anything you want. "I am safe", "I can do this", "I am strong", "It will work out". If you have time, a shower, bath, long meditation, music, candles - anything can work - just let it be you for a while. A clearer calmer mind will help you to be able to see solutions and work things out with more focus and clarity.

ॐ Nighttime Meditation ॐ

As we know, with M.E. sleep can be all or nothing. Even after a 12 hour sleep, you awake feeling as though you've been awake for a week. Other times you're not sleeping at all. It doesn't matter how many hours you sleep, it's never enough. You're physically and emotionally drained and unable to function.

Insomnia can also be a problem. Awake when you should be sleep. Counting the hours. Hearing the clock tick in the dark. While everyone else is happily sleeping, you're awake staring at the ceiling. Whatever your sleep patterns, it can be depressing and frustrating for both M.E. warriors and people that care for them.

Now you are wondering how yoga can help with getting a restful peaceful sleep?

Well, yoga as we now know doesn't just work on the body, it helps the mind as well. A calm mind is a good starting point when needing a good rest. Yoga and breath-work help calm the nervous system, which in turn sends calm signals to the muscles and brain to say it's ok to relax, helping you to slowly drift off to sleep.

Here are a few tips and a visualization method that, with practice can help your sleep feel more restful.

First, make sure your bed is fresh, comfortable and not too cold or hot. We spend a huge portion of our time in there so let's see and think of bed as the most comfortable place ever. Try not to excite your brain with too much TV, thrilling books or movies just before bed. You want your body and mind to be calm and quiet. Pick the same time every night to start meditation which will help to establish a sleep pattern. Slowly your mind and body will start to know when it's meditation and bedtime. Don't try and force sleep. The more you think and try, the more of a fight your body and mind will give you. Don't give up either. Quieting the mind is a tough exercise, it will take time.

If you're struggling and getting frustrated, breathe deeper. Focus on the sound of your breath. Create a picture in your mind or repeat a mantra until you can feel relaxed again.

Visualization meditation and breathing techniques go hand in hand. They will calmly and naturally rest your body.

Get comfortable lying on your back. Legs relaxed and arms either by your side, or placed gently on your stomach to feel the breath. See Savasana (page 45). Focus on your breathing. Take 10 deep slow breaths. You can use counting to help you focus, for example counting to 4 on an inhale and 4 on an exhale. You can also focus gently on the rising and falling of your stomach if your hands are placed there. Spend a few minutes here, slowing your breath down.

Once you start to feel relaxed, close your eyes and picture yourself in your favourite place. It could be a beach, by a lake, in a field of flowers, by a waterfall. Somewhere outside with an abundance of fresh air.

Wherever you are, it's warm and sunny. You're alone, with only nature's sounds around you. You soak up the warm feeling that's surrounding you, like an invisible blanket. The sun slowly begins to relax all your muscles and you feel your aches slowly melt away. You feel free, healthy and calm. A smile comes softly across your face. Explore your surroundings. Sit and listen to the birds. Watch the clouds. Stop here for as long as you want soaking up the surroundings, sounds and warmth. This is your happy place. Don't give up if you struggle to keep the focus while meditating. It's too easy for thoughts to pop up in the mind or worries, doubts and tasks. You can't stop these thoughts coming into your mind, but with practice you can simply not react to them. See them, and then see them float, pop or be washed away in your scene or place of peace. Stay here until you feel yourself drifting to sleep.

ॐ Questions & Answers ॐ

Exercise is supposed to be avoided with M.E. How is yoga different?

Yoga is a balance of mind, body and spirit. It`s only recently been famed for its high powered workouts for the lean bodies that we constantly see. Power yoga is a "no go" for M.E. sufferers as it`s cardio based. Restorative, gentle yoga, along with proper breathing techniques, can help balance, detox and strengthen muscles and body organs, while the deep breathing helps circulate oxygen and fresh blood to cells, lungs and brain helping our immune and central nervous system to work more effectively.

I did yoga before & it left me with a flare up. How can I avoid this again?

Yoga comes in a variety of forms. Make sure if you`re going to a class that it`s for beginners, restorative or specially tailored to meet your needs. Don't try to "keep up" with others. Listen to your body. If a pose says to be held for 5 breaths, hold it for 2 and slowly build up over time. If you`re doing it from home, start with 5 minutes' practice with sitting or lying poses. See and note how you feel after. Build up the time to hold the poses and then add more time to your practice slowly. Some days, with M.E. its 2 steps forward and 5 back, so on the days where you don't feel well, focus on meditation or 1 or 2 gentle poses from your bed. Don't over push your body. Start with yoga once a week, then add more time. You can also start with 1 pose slowly adding another each week. M.E.

is an up and down illness. Yoga can be adapted to suit the illness and your needs.

What is the best way to start yoga?

Find out what you are wanting from yoga. Is it for physical, mental or emotional needs. Did you want to help muscles and joint pain? Or to try calm a restless mind? Then find a pose which is suited to your needs and wants. Take 5 minutes out of your day to practise this 1 pose. Breathe deeply while focusing your mind on how this pose is making your body and mind feel. Start with a gentle short routine if you wish. Just avoid long DVD`s or "full workouts" which can cause more harm than health.

M.E. leaves me bed-bound for long periods of time. Can I still do yoga?

Yes. Yoga isn't always about standing up and standing on your head. Yoga can be done even as you lie down in bed. Start by focusing on breathing work and meditation for bad days. This helps to bring blood and oxygen to the body. Then introduce 2 poses a day. 1 in the morning to help open your body to help relieve and prevent stiffness and 1 pose for the evening to help relax body and mind. Hold the poses for as long as is comfortable to you. Gradually build up the time you hold the pose, or add a new pose / change the poses.

Do I need to buy anything specific to practise yoga?

Not at all. I designed this yoga so that you can do it in the comfort of your pjs. It's also designed so that it can be done on your bed. However, if you wish you can purchase a yoga mat and the workouts can be done on the floor or outside. Dressing gown straps can be used to help align the poses, and deepen the stretch if you wish. Cushions or pillows can be added to rest your head or under the buttocks to help forward folds. All things which you can find around your home.

ॐ Closing Notes ॐ

We all have 2 choices of how we look at things in our life. The good side or the bad. I saw the bad regarding M.E. for a long time, but with all that me time and as I grew older and not so much wiser, I learnt to see this illness as an opportunity for personal growth. It was my teacher, my guide and as it worked out it also became part of my life's purpose.

It's a time we can spend learning about ourselves, to evaluate our life, our choices, our true happiness. To discover who we are and what we want in life and find our best path on the road to recovery. I'm not going to say it's easy or a short journey, but it is well worth experiencing self-discovery. Accept where you are now and what is happening. Come to terms with the illness if you can. We suffer more if we hold on to anger, trying to keep up with a busy (normal) life, in denial about the things we can't do anymore. Our energy is used up by us struggling, and we as M.E. warriors know that energy is very precious to us. As stress is the most common cause of exhaustion, let it go. We can only move forward and see the new horizon if we let go of the past, let go of what we can't change and all the built up negative emotions that are stored in our precious body.

Something new, something better, something exciting is waiting to happen. Listen to your inner guidance. Accept the limitations you have at the moment and work with them. You may never get back your previous lifestyle, but you'll have a better, more peaceful lifestyle. I still work around M.E. with regards to the hours and days which I work. Sometimes it's all too easy to fit a client in here or there on a day off or first thing in the morning because it's a better time for them, but it's not better for my health and that's my number one priority. So work with the M.E. instead of against it and it can work alongside you and what you want to do with your life.

I hope this book has given you some hope and a new love for yoga. I hope the yoga has helped with your muscle aches and pains as it has helped me on numerous occasions. Don't get discouraged with the poses or more importantly yourself. You are a beautiful, strong and capable being and I believe in you, so please believe in yourself too.

Namaste.

ॐ Testimonials ॐ

I am very excited to see *Yoga, My Bed & M.E.* encouraging M.E. sufferers. Take a look at what this lady is doing. Far better than anything the NHS has ever offered me in my 12 years' experience as a patient.   - Nikki

Absolutely loving my yoga journey and couldn't have done this without Donna. Thank you so much. I finally feel like I am doing something worthwhile to help my recovery.
- Amy

Donna is so sweet and supportive. She has M.E./CFS and anxiety. What I love is that she is adapting yoga to our level. When you look online, the fitness routines are too hard for us. We try them, fail and give up. Sometimes we can`t get out of bed other days we can stretch, so I thought I would learn from someone who understands us. – Mel

I`ve tried and failed with exercise until I was introduced to this yoga programme by *Yoga, My Bed & M.E.* It`s been a blessing. It eases the discomfort in my muscles, soothes my stomach and keeps me calm and rested. I am sleeping better, and I feel more positive too. It is easy and gentle, which is what my body needs. M.E. patients should look into *Yoga, My Bed & M.E* yoga programmes. – Jemma

ॐ Acknowledgements ॐ

I would like to dedicate this book to my illness. Without it being my teacher I wouldn't be who and where I am today.

I dedicate it to every person reading this book. You are strong, beautiful and never stop shining. The world needs you.

I would like to thank my rock, my mum for having to put up with me and M.E. For her continued help and support through the roller coaster of my life.

Thank you to my daughter, Mollie. You kept me going and made me stronger. Your smile makes everything better and thank you for having the patience of a saint and being the best, most beautiful daughter anyone could wish for.

Thank you to my best friend, Paul, who over the past years has supported, listened and been there to make me smile when I didn't feel like smiling.

A massive thank you to Mike for taking the great pictures and being a longtime supportive friend and to Sheila, who encouraged me to write and who took time to help with my book.

Thank you all from the bottom of my heart. I am truly grateful.

ॐ **Disclaimer** ॐ

Before starting any new form of exercise it`s advisable to seek medical guidance and advice from your doctors or specialists.

The information given in this book shouldn't be treated as a substitute for any professional medical advice.

Donna Owens and *Yoga, My Bed & M.E.* hold no responsibilities for any injuries, illnesses, loss, claims, damage or, at worst death from taking part in this yoga programme. The yoga in this book is done at the reader`s own responsibility and own risk.

No part of this book may be reproduced or copied without written permission.

ॐ About Donna ॐ

Donna is constantly updating her qualifications in yoga and health.

She has already gained: Yoga in Health Level 3 and Anatomy and Physiology Distinction Level 3

She studied M.E / CFS recovery and is looking to add more nutrition, yoga and health qualifications to her CV.

www.donnayogagirl.com is where you can find her very popular guides:

- ✓ Restful Mind & Muscles Bedtime Yoga Guide
- ✓ Yoga for Anxiety & Stress
- ✓ Yoga for M.E. Flare Up Days
- ✓ Simple Yoga for M.E.

to download and carry out the yoga from your phone or tablet.

More guides are being planned for 2017, along with Donna`s You Tube Channel: *Yoga, My Bed & M.E.*

Donna is also planning her second book.

ॐ **Notes** ॐ

Here you can jot down details of times, days and how you felt to measure your yoga progress. This will help you find the best yoga times and poses to work for you.

ॐ **Notes** ॐ

ॐ **Index of Poses** ॐ

"What you do today to help aid recovery sets the path for your future." – Donna Owens.